Torrance Hates SMA

Torrance Johnson and the Johnson Family

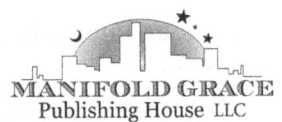

Torrance Hates SMA
Copyright (C) 2013 Torrance and Katrina Johnson

All rights reserved. No part of this book may be copied or reproduced in any form without written permission from the publisher.

Photographs:
Cover courtesy of Ms. Enre Laney, shot on location at the TLAB Accelerated Learning Center in Detroit World Outreach Church
Michelle Obama Photos courtesy of The White House
MDA Lock-Up courtesy of Ms. Karen D. Hollins, *I on You Photography*
Cover design: CreativeLogoArt

Story Compilation: as told to Darlene Carol Dickson and written by Torrance Johnson and the Johnson family

ISBN: 978-1-937400-29-3
ISBN: 978-1-937400-30-9 ebook

Printed in the United States of America

Published by Manifold Grace Publishing House, LLC
Southfield, Michigan 48033
www.manifoldgracepublishinghouse.com

Dedication

To all the kids in wheelchairs

In memory of Grandma Edith Johnson
To Grandma Evelyn Kirk
To Grandpa Booker T. Johnson

Acknowledgments

Thank you to my Mom and Dad who are always there for me. Also to my sisters Areon and Tionna and my brother Lavonta.

Thank you to Ms. Darlene for working with me.

Last, but not least, thank you to Eriksson Elementary School in Canton, Michigan.

Table of Contents

	Dedication	v
	Acknowledgments	vii
	Forewords	xi
	Introduction	xvii
1.	Just Like Everyone Else	1
2.	Welcome to My World	3
3.	Family Time	7
4.	My Mom Speaks	13
5.	Highlights	25
6.	A Hope and a Future	33
7.	MDA Letter	35
8.	About the Authors	37

Forewords

On January 14, 2006, God blessed Torrance and Katrina Johnson with a baby boy – Torrance Johnson Jr., the pride of their life. In December 2008, Torrance Jr. was diagnosed with Spinal Muscular Atrophy Type 2, a disease that is terminal and progressive. With this disease, the motor neuron affects the voluntary muscles that are used for activities such as crawling, walking, head and neck control and the ability to swallow. This rare disorder affects approximately 1 in every 6,000 babies born in the United States. Because of the prayer life of Mr. and Mrs. Johnson and the support of their church family, little Torrance enjoys a normal active lifestyle. He is very involved in the youth program as a leader and is very outspoken in every situation.

Little Torrance is in command of his wheel chair, able to go anywhere he likes to go at any speed. He refuses to let this disease take control of his life. Little Torrance is a poster boy for this disease. My prayer for him is that he lives his life to the glory of God.

Pastor John O. Wright Jr.
New Hope Church of the Nazarene
February 16, 2014

\\

Almost eight year old Torrance E. Johnson Jr. is beautiful. He has big brown eyes, an intelligent face, and a huge smile. Torrance is outgoing and happy, he loves life, he's crazy smart, loves to meet new people, and has zero fear of speaking in public. Torrance is one of the coolest kids you'll ever meet.

But Torrance E. Johnson Jr. has a disease that can kill him. It's called Spinal Muscular Atrophy or SMA for short. SMA is a form of muscular dystrophy. It is progressive and fatal and robs those who have it of the ability to run, to walk, to swallow, to breathe. There is no cure; not yet.

SMA is only part of who Torrance is. SMA doesn't stop this amazing young man from living fully, from opening his arms and his heart to helping and inspiring others. Torrance has been selected as the MDA's Michigan Goodwill Ambassador for 2014. Torrance has two parents, two older sisters, and an older brother who love him very much. He goes to camp, he swims, he plays video games. Torrance is full of love and life. But SMA has taken so much. It's robbed him of his ability to walk so he uses a powerchair. A machine helps Torrance breathe easier at night, a feeding tube provides nutrients while he sleeps and other machines help him to cough and clear secretions when he's sick. SMA is an ugly, evil disease.

I met Torrance in 2009 and I love him. His mother is my best friend. She understands what it's like to raise a child with a catastrophic disease. She understands how important this young man is. She knows what she must do to keep him alive, and she does it with love and grace. The world is a better place because of this wonderful, sweet boy and Katrina, his fighter mom.

Love,
Wendy Persinger
January 4, 2014

I was with Torrance and Katrina when Little Torrance was born. He came into this world looking handsome and healthy. Shortly after being born the nurses said they would have to take him to the pediatric intensive care unit, just for observation. All appeared to be well. After coming home, and as time progressed, there seemed to be challenges that Torrance was experiencing, which Katrina and Torrance later shared would be a diagnosis of Spinal Muscular Atrophy (SMA).

Of course, I was shocked. I didn't understand, so how could they as his parents. This was distressing news that I didn't want to admit. More importantly, I knew I had to become educated regarding what was happening with Little Torrance. I had to be able to communicate effectively with his parents regarding what was happening to their child and the family, as a result of this disease.

I'm sure the family was scared, confused, didn't understand, questioned why them and probably had many, many more questions, concerns and emotions. However, in observing the kids you would never know that anything was different with Torrance, other than them providing him assistance and love, when and where needed. The parents were visibly shaken upon first learning and trying to understand, but as time passed, they became stronger and stronger. Their faith increased, they became advocates for their son and the SMA organization. Tears turned into smiles and they are thankful for this marvelous son that they have in Torrance.

Now, Little Torrance...I have never in life met a child such as him. Clearly, he is special. I believe he is chosen by God to show his family, friends and all those he comes in contact with how to live, face life threatening challenges, and yet be courageous, strong with an unshakeable foundation in Christ. In spite of his limitations, setbacks and challenges he is a leader in all areas of his life, and sets the example for all. This entire family is special! I thank God I'm allowed to be a part of such a remarkable family structure.

Pastor Marie A. Williams
January 12, 2014

\~

A very good friend told me about a young woman she met who had a 7 year old son who wanted to write a book. This was very intriguing; however it took me several weeks before contacting Katrina Johnson, the child's mother. The culprit was simply time and involvement in previous and current projects that were about to end. In any case, I did contact Katrina and after some conversation, set up a meeting.

Several things impressed me and yes, my initial impressions were correct; I was intrigued. First of all, Torrance was delightful. He had a really big personality that exceeded his wheelchair. There was something immediately engaging in his smile, something a bit mischievous. I noticed right away that he had jokes about each of his family members; his dad in particular.

Mom was truly the 'hall monitor' as it were. She settled Torrance when he went too far out on a limb. She watched as he ate, she told his story when necessary; she was acutely tuned in to all aspects of his care. Actually, the whole family was. If he cleared his throat, they all glanced with an alertness that would allow them to react if he didn't right himself.

This told me that, while Torrance was in the chair - the one with the issue - the whole family was affected. This whole blended family cared for Torrance and cared about Torrance. And he cared about them. He can't rough house with his dad or brother, but he can 'rough house' with his wit and humor.

After Torrance told me about the book he wanted to write and explained how and what SMA was, I sent the family off to write the book. And after several interviews and collecting the pieces they wrote, compiling their work was easy as the family was very transparent; often painfully so. I believe in young Torrance and his desire to help and inspire other families like his. I believe in his vision and his hope and his joy and his desire to be free from the disease. And I just know you will too when you read this book. You will truly understand why *Torrance Hates SMA*. And I hate it too!

Darlene Carol Dickson
CEO, Manifold Grace Publishing House, LLC
November 22, 2013

Introduction

My name is Torrance Johnson Jr. and I wanted to write a book so that parents and kids know what to look forward to or experience when the kids have SMA or MD (Muscular Dystrophy). SMA is Spinal Muscular Atrophy and I understand it to be a disabling disease that prevents kids from walking and causes them to have breathing problems and problems with their muscles. My doctors make me feel happy because they understand what I'm going through and they help me understand it better. Dr. McCormick and my mom explain it to me where a kid can understand it.

SMA Type II is a neuro-muscular disease that is a terminal and progressive disease. It affects all of the nerves and muscles in the body.

When I was 3 years old I was diagnosed with Spinal Muscular Atrophy. My family and I were very sad. I felt good that I knew what I had, but sad that I could barely walk. And I could not run with my friends. Sometimes I feel scared because I don't know why I was picked for this disease.

Sometimes I feel bad because my muscles are so weak and I really wish God would help me walk. But, I have a strong mind and even though I have a disease, I don't let it affect me.

I chose the book title because it is from my heart. I

hate what it does to my body.

1. Just Like Everyone Else

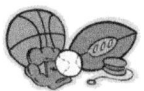

I love school. I go to Eriksson Elementary School which is a great school. They don't judge me because I am in a wheelchair. I'm not the only kid in a wheelchair. The other kid's name is Jonathan. My favorite subjects are science and math and my specials are art, music, gym, library and computer.

I get asked a lot "Why are you in a chair?" "Why are you not up walking?" Some people think that it is cool to have a person around in a wheelchair. Sometimes it's fun being in a chair – until I can't run and play like other kids.

School was hard when I first went because people didn't understand why I was in a chair. They treated me differently because they were scared. They asked me if it was easy getting around and I replied "No, because I can't walk around like everyone else!" Then they made comments like "Poor thing, you have to be in that chair" or "I wish I had one of those chairs." That used to make me put my head down and feel sad. But now I say "Well, what if you woke up tomorrow and you could not walk?"

That usually shuts them up. If you don't have anything nice to say, don't say anything at all. But now I'm in a school where they get it. They don't treat me like I'm in a wheelchair. I'm just like everyone else.

2. Welcome to My World

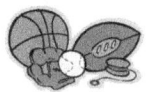

I've been in a chair since I was 3 years old. Most people with SMA have been in a chair since they were babies, our disability is permanent. I also have lots of machines I have to use. There is a vest, feeding tube, cough assist, nebulizer, suction machine, and BiPap machine. They help with feeding problems and help clear my lungs.

The BiPap is a machine that puts mist into my lungs to make them expand. I put it over my nose and it wraps around my head. I don't like this machine because it is very uncomfortable. I used to cry when I first got it. On occasion I still cry, even if I'm in the hospital and get admitted and have to use it. My mom tells the doctors and they deliver it to my room. I hate it altogether whether at home or the hospital.

Having to be on the machines also stops me from having fun. I remember one time my cousin Damon came over and I could not play with him because I had to be on the machine. I felt bad about that, he is like a brother and a best friend to me. Another time I went to Damon's house to play in the water. The water was really cold, so my uncle hooked the hose up to the hot water in the house to make the water warm enough for me to play in. I love him for that because I cannot play in regular cold water like everyone else. My bones get very bad in cold water and I can't move. My mom has to get me out.

Not everything is bad about having SMA. I started public speaking when I was 5 years old. My cousin attends Oakland Community College and she did a paper on my disease. Then her class wanted to know more about it and about me so it was the first time I did public speaking. I explained to them how I use my power chair and I told them about my five machines and feeding tube. I even told them about my fight with my school.

The school did not want to give me an aide. They also said I could not take my machines into school because it would take up too much time. There were problems with that school.

My last day at that school was in May, 2012. My Mom and Dad were upset because while I was in my manual wheelchair, a kid was pushing me and there was a hill in front of the school. I went rolling down that hill. I tried to reach for my brakes, but could not; so I rolled right into a parked car. My face was hurting, my front tooth got knocked out and my lip was busted. Mom came and took me to Urgent Care. They gave me Motrin for my headache and told my Mom to keep an eye on me. Well, my head kept hurting.

Two days later my Mom took me back to the doctor who said I suffered a mild concussion. I felt bad. Now I don't have to worry about the old school anymore since we moved from Detroit to Canton because I kept getting hurt. Like one time the driver of my bus didn't strap me in my chair. Now I don't have to worry about getting hurt at school, falling off the toilet or out of my chair.

I am really looking forward to summer camp! This will be my first year. I have heard so many stories of how kids ride horses, motorcycles and eat ice cream all day. All the kids have a helper and I'm very excited because some of my friends are going to be there. But the only thing is, I have to take those machines with me for 6 days. Welcome to my world.

Torrance Hates SMA

3. Family Time

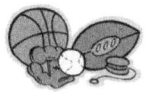

I love my family. My parents are great and I have two sisters and one brother. Their names are Areon, Lavonta and Tionna. My brother and sisters help me all the time.

Lavonta helps me when I'm in my bed and I'm trying to get something off the floor; he gets it for me. Areon is good to talk to when I'm sad or mad. Tionna plays with me and helps me if I need something and I can't reach it. She taught me how to write in cursive.

I feel like my power chair, "Blue Jay" is part of the family too. He helps me get around. When I first got him, I was so happy that no one had to push me around any longer. I was independent.

And now I would like for you to meet my family.

Dad

On January 14, 2006 Torrance Elton Johnson Jr., my son, was born. My wife had a normal pregnancy. She had made all doctor appointments and did the things necessary to have Torrance naturally. That day was so exciting and peaceful. I was glad that he was coming. He was the one gift I prayed for, a son. I love my daughter Tionna, but I would love to have a chance to correct the things I thought were wrong in me – through him. God gave me what I wanted. I talked and played with my son every chance I got and I knew he was going to be different from the other kids.

As he grew, I thought everything was okay with him. But when he walked, he fell down a lot. I didn't know he wasn't able to walk. At that time I thought he was just taking his time. At the age of 3 we found out he had Spinal Muscular Atrophy.

I didn't know anything about this disease. But I quickly found out it was a disease that would cause him to be in a wheelchair and very weak. My heart was heavy, didn't understand why this was happening. I am a believer in Christ and I said that all my children are His and whatever God has for them, so be it.

I'm not saying I didn't get upset and lash out about my youngest child not being able to do all the physical things I thought he would do when he got older. But, I had to accept the situation and deal with it.

Physically, Torrance Jr. isn't able to do much but mentally, my son has the ability to do whatever he puts his mind to. Sometimes it gets hard and I get upset, but when I think about it, he is just a normal little boy who enjoys his parents, siblings and friends. He is a light; a friend who is more caring than most of us adults. What some see as a disability, he views it as a way to show that it's okay to be different. I'm very proud of my son.

Torrance Elton Johnson Sr.

Big Sister

In 2008, my brother was diagnosed with SMA (Spinal Muscular Atrophy). It is a terminal illness that attacks your spine, and weakens it where you're not able to walk. We (my family and I) knew, before he was diagnosed, that he was different than other babies. When he started walking, he would take a couple of steps and then fall on the floor.

As he got older, he took less and less steps until he could no longer walk. In 2010, he needed the assistance of multiple machines to help him survive. As the years passed he needed the use of a wheelchair or the help from my family and me to be mobile.

My experience with my brother has been a roller coaster ride. It has its ups mostly, but some downs too. It is a struggle that my family and I go through dealing with my brother's disease. It has been hard on us from the beginning. It is hard for me to go to sleep sometimes, knowing that the same person I love and have fun with could be gone at any moment. To be honest, I don't know what I would do if he was gone. We are so close that my whole world would be upside down. But I still have to live every day for myself and not as if he was going to die.

Last year he reached a milestone; he turned 6 years old. This year he is 7. On the outside he is brilliant, articulate, well-dressed and strong; but on the inside, the older he gets, the weaker he gets. The challenge I face is as the sister of a boy who is a son, who is a brother, who is a nephew and who could be gone out of our lives forever; and I can't do anything about it.

This isn't a challenge in my life that I have overcome. It is going to be ongoing until my brother is gone to heaven. I am happy that I am not alone. I have my parents and my other two siblings to help me with my daily struggle. All I can do is keep hope and faith that my brother stays here to live his life like everyone else. I feel that I must keep the faith, knowing that eventually he will be with God.

We have a weird unspeakable bond,
My love for him goes to infinity and beyond
Even though he is still like a flower that has to grow
He is wise and has patience - you will never know

Areon Kirk

Brother

Hi, my name is Lavonta Dilliard and I'm Torrance Johnson's brother. I am 13 years old and I go to East Middle School. I get good grades and am very active.

My brother Torrance is very nice and he is very smart like his dad. I feel bad that he has this disease. I feel sad because when Torrance wants to walk, he can't. I believe there is a reason for everything, so I think that God put Torrance on earth to spread peace and joy; also so he could change lives all over the world.

When people look at him like he is an alien or something, I get mad. So if you see him, don't just look at him all crazy, talk to him! Ask him questions or just smile. After all the things that Torrance goes through and the stuff people may say or do, he is still happy to be alive. He has faith that there will be a cure for this disease and I do too.

Every night I tell him "I love you bro," because we never know what is going to happen or when it will. But at the end of the day, when he is happy, I am happy.

Lavonta Dilliard

Little Sister

My Feelings About Torrance

- When Torrance was first born he was a cute baby. He was 8 pounds and 13 ounces. He was 2 when he got diagnosed with SMA. When he was 3 he ran into our brand new TV; it broke. At age 6 he was very smart in school. That's when we had a make-over at our old house. We came home and it looked nicer than ever before. And when he turned 7, it was a milestone.

  His party was fun. He had Smiley the Clown and there was a lot of food. We had to take some home. After that we went home to go to sleep. The next day I woke up and fell on the ground, I was so tired.

- Sometimes I am still sad because people make fun of Torrance and stare at him. Sometimes I just want to punch them in the face but I ignore them and keep going. One day this boy at school said he felt sorry for Torrance. I had to straight face him and told him, "Don't be, he's just like you!" It was pretty obvious he was not going to listen to me; he just stood there and looked at me like I was stupid. I looked at him the same way. I was pretty sure he thought I was crazy, but that's okay.

- Yesterday Torrance had a doctor's appointment so I didn't have anything to write.

- My brother likes my friend Sarah but my friends Katie, Morgan and Shannon like to chase him around when we play outside at recess. I always catch him at a bad time because he always runs over my foot with his wheelchair!

- In May my Gramma died. I was so sad, so was Torrance. But I was the one who was crying the most, I couldn't even go to school for a day. I just didn't want to deal with the other kids, some kids are mean. But I didn't want Torrance to see me all mushy, so I tried to suck it up because I'm older than him and I want to show a good example.

- One night I had a dream that Torrance died. I talked to my mom about it and she said "It's nothing but the devil." I never want to see my brother die because I'll be mad at myself because I did not spend enough time with him. I love my little brother. I know I'm nine but he's kind of like an older brother sometimes.

I love Torrance.

Tionna Johnson

4. My Mom Speaks

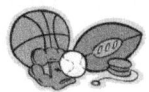

The Year That Changed My Life

When I got pregnant in April 2005 it was pure joy. My husband and I were excited to be having a boy. It was a gift from God. After a couple of months, people commented that I was glowing. It was a good pregnancy, I felt better than I had my whole life; peaceful, no worries.

On January 14, 2006 at 7:00p.m., I gave birth to Torrance Jr. He was 8 lbs. 13 oz., a big boy. We were overjoyed and felt blessed. From birth to between four to six months he passed all of his milestones, but he was not independent. He was not sitting up or crawling. Not until his first birthday did he try standing. After two steps he fell immediately. And after a few days of the same thing happening and because of the leg pain, he was walking with a limp.

I called his pediatrician who watched him fall after a few steps but said I was being overprotective. It still didn't seem right to me so I asked for an MRI and finally got it. Then I took him to Children's Hospital where they sent him to physical therapy and said something was wrong, but they didn't know what.

I took my baby to over six different hospitals; they

all said he would be okay. Finally I found the Michigan Institute for Neurological Disorders in the yellow pages and within two weeks we were in for blood tests. On a Tuesday in December 2008 my 2 ½ year old son tested positive for a disease called Spinal Muscular Atrophy Type II. This would explain the leg pain, the falling and the weakness all over his body. When the doctor, Dr. Eileen McCormick, gave us the results, I cried. I felt as if I had been shot.

What do I do now? Why didn't I find out sooner? How will I explain this to people? Can I care for him and my other children? WHY ME? I immediately went home and called family and friends.

I hadn't felt so bad since I tragically found my mother dead in 1994. And even though I had the strength of God that time, this was different. From 2007 through 2012 I went through a deep depression. This disease began to define where I went, who came around us, when I was happy or sad. I had absolutely no control of what was going on. I tried shopping my problems away, I tried going to church but no one could understand what we were going through.

The Family Effect

I got into arguments with my husband because I would continually buy toys for Torrance. My husband would always tell me, "It's in God's hands." I would argue back with him, "I know that but I need God to fix him!"

My husband would sometimes have to leave work to come home and comfort me because I was such a mess. I would go into the bathroom to get myself together while he talked to the day care kids.

Who could I call and talk to, who would understand? All I could say is "Lord, help me!" Now, while all of this was going on, my house was not handicapped accessible. I had that to worry about and there was no equity in our home for renovations. All the doors seemed to be closing in on us, but my husband would always say, "God's got us."

"How can you say that when the whole world is falling down around us?"
"That's all I know," he'd answer.

I was mad that he went to work. I was mad that he felt like this. I was just mad and I felt all alone. I'd had enough and I wanted him to leave. I wanted to be free. "Let's separate. I can't go on like this."

He would just look at me with hurt in his eyes, "You don't mean it!"
"Yes, I do. If we separate for a while we can clear our heads, then we can get back together." So I thought.

I was pretty sure I did not want to be married any longer. I just wanted to separate from him and focus on my baby. What did my husband know anyway? I was the one up in the middle of the night putting him on feeding machines and breathing machines. He just went to work every day – I felt like all I needed him for was financial support. I wasn't even sure I liked or loved him anymore. How could I? I had to focus every minute of every day helping my son. Who could think about other things at a time like that? In the meantime, my family was suffering. My young kids did not have me – I gave all my attention to Torrance. I knew I had to get myself together. It didn't help that in 2012 my husband, who was already diabetic, found out that his kidneys were failing.

I also figured out a way to mend things with him since he never agreed that we should separate. We learned that my problems are his problems and vice versa. On June 8, 2013 he asked me to remarry him and I said yes. Together we all deal with Torrance's issues.

My Baby Boy

With his loss of appetite and constant pneumonia (every six weeks) they immediately ordered breathing machines and a wheel chair so he could be independent. They also ordered a bathing chair. He got so much new equipment in that first year that I cried every time the doorbell rang and a new piece of equipment was delivered.

But why did he have to have five machines AND a feeding tube? "Lord, help my son breathe!" God said "I give you breath every morning." When he got the feeding tube and I prayed about it God said "I gave you my word which is the bread of life. You will never want as long as you keep faith in me." I cried even more, if that was possible, then I went on a fast, read my bible, taught Sunday School. I just wanted to get God's attention so He would heal my child.

It didn't help that Torrance was having trouble in school. In 2009, he was in preschool. They were glad to have him and he was glad to be there. It seemed like a nice school. They had kids with and without special needs. But was that good enough for Torrance? He was different. He could not get out of the chair by himself, could not feed himself. And they often thought he was strong enough to do certain things his body would not allow him to do. So, NO, they did not understand Torrance's needs.

I asked my doctor from the Michigan Institute for Neurological Disorders to speak with the school and they did. Prior to this he had an accident where he fell while sitting on the toilet. I believe they thought they understood the care Torrance needed, but they did not. I cried because they just didn't get it.

Every time they called me from his school, which was more than five times, I would pick him up and keep him home with me. This was my son who was ill and I wanted him to be happy. Also, this might be my last time with him and I felt like this for years.

Then the doctors also thought Torrance had neuroblastoma, a cancer that attacks the nerves in children. After testing him, thankfully, the results came back negative. There were so many situations or issues we had to deal with regarding this SMA. Because the school he went to was uneducated about the disease, they treated him like kids with no disability. For example the toilet incident; because his back is weak, it can give out at any time and he can fall off the toilet. That is just what happened, he fell and hit his ear and the side of his face. It bruised badly.

The teacher said he didn't know what happened. He'd just closed the door and went to the entrance of the restroom when he heard a loud thump and "I fell".

First of all, why was his teacher helping him? Why didn't he have a para-pro? It seems Detroit Public Schools (DPS) could not afford it, even though the teacher was not medically qualified. I just wanted my child safe so I met with his teachers. He had four at the time. We tried to schedule a meeting with the principal but she was never available.

There were two other times where Torrance fell out of a chair they put him in instead of leaving him in his wheelchair. Another time he was on the bus and fell because the driver did not strap him in. I called the principal both times to let her know what happened and so she would be aware that DPS bus transportation was the worst ever for Torrance. Unfortunately, all I could do was call and complain. We did not have a vehicle to transport him and his wheelchair in.

One night I was talking to my son and he said, "Mommy, are you okay?"
I answered him, "Yes".
"Then why are you crying?"
I told him it was because I loved him so much.
He said, "I love you too. Every night I talk to God, don't be afraid Mommy."
I left the room after that, crying on my way out.

That night God spoke to me and said, "If I wanted to I could take your son right now. You can't buy his time from me, I make all things happen. I could just snap my fingers, but I have something for him to do - so get yourself together." From that day forward I stopped all the shopping and helped him discover his calling. He said he wanted to speak to people and make them feel better. Every night he would write in his notebook.

One day Torrance was talking to one of his teachers who had been mean to him. He said "I forgive you" and he wanted to pray with her. They were not supposed to, but they prayed together and she later said he made her feel good every time she saw him.

Before long we got a call from the MDA (Muscular Dystrophy Association). They wanted Torrance to speak to a high school class about his disease. I asked Torrance about it and he said "Sure". Well, he went and spoke and there was not a dry eye in the place. They said he spoke very well and answered all their questions. Even the teacher was in tears. Torrance goes out every chance he gets and speaks to college students and others about the disease and his life. He says "I was born to be a public speaker!"

Torrance was still like any other child and wanted to be around other children. He would pray too. He would call me to pray when he woke up and when he went to bed. He took his bible with him everywhere and talked to the kids at school about God. When he said he wanted to speak to people and make them feel better I wasn't ready for it. But when he got invites to speak, and I didn't think I could do it, he would say "God told me to speak to people and share about my disease and help people feel good."

"But, I don't know how to speak in front of people."
He simply said "Just drive me there and I'll do all of the talking. I hear you say you want God to heal me, but I told God 'if you don't heal me I'll still serve you. Either way I'll serve you with all my heart.' I'm not

letting this disease hold me back."

I decided enough was enough. If he can fight this, then I can too. No more pity party. I remember my aunt saying, "When the devil wants to fight, you don't back down; you put on your boxing gloves and say come on, let's dance devil!" I started praying before we left home and feeding myself positive thoughts.

Now we're living one day at a time. Torrance is 8 years old and doing well. He still uses all of his machines for respiratory help and he still needs help bathing, toileting, getting dressed and feeding. He is an excellent student, getting all A's in school and acting as the teacher's helper. She says he is always helping someone else.

Torrance has an active life. He is a public speaker, he sings and ushers at church. Having his own shoe line called 'Toe Jams' for Exceptional Kids is just one of his dreams. Some days are better than others but it has brought our family closer together. He likes the words of the song, *"My good days outweigh my bad days, I say thank you Lord, I won't complain."*

I think we, our family, are learning how to deal with and cope with this issue. It is a battle every day, it is a struggle.

In 2012 Torrance told me he wanted a lot of pictures to remember people by. I asked him "why"? He told me "I just need a lot of pictures for when I leave". My heart was shattered into a thousand pieces. Now me, not thinking into the future, thought he meant right now. Anyway, I took a deep breath and spoke to some folks about pictures. For his 6th birthday we had everyone bring a picture of themselves.

Throughout this whole time I've learned a lot. I learned how to fight for my son no matter what! I am his voice. I learned how to stand up to doctors and teachers for Torrance's best interests. I also learned about Torrance's disease. True enough I used to cry every chance I got, but on January 14th every year, I know it is not about me.

This kid had a mission and he was going to do it whether I agreed or not. I had to pull myself together for him; to join him on his mission. He loves to write and I started writing. It helps us to heal our pain. No more eating through my depression all the time.

I dislike the fact that we can't travel out of town without all of his machines but I'm a super mom and he is a super kid. We won't let anything hold us back!

Welcome to Our Day

Some of the equipment Torrance uses on a daily basis includes:

- Ramp
- Wheelchair
- Walker
- Stroller
- Cough Assist
- Helmet
- Vest Machine
- BiPap Machine
- Bath Chair
- Nebulizer

- Feeding Tube
- Suction Machine
- Braces
- Stander
- Lifter (for the van)

I like that SMA:	I hate that SMA:
<ul><li>Makes him outspoken</li><li>Makes him optimistic</li><li>Makes him courageous</li><li>Makes him a fighter</li><li>Makes him strong-willed</li><li>Makes him hopeful, confident, bright, caring, humble</li><li>Strengthens his faith in God</li><li>Brings the family together</li><li>Introduces us to new people going through the same journey</li><li>Helps you find strength you didn't know you had</li></ul>	<ul><li>Lessens his ability to walk, run, ride bikes etc.</li><li>Causes him to be on 6 machines</li><li>Causes him to be in a wheelchair</li><li>Requires a special vehicle</li><li>Causes people to give him strange looks</li><li>Causes people to be afraid to touch him</li><li>IS A DISEASE THAT CAN KILL HIM</li></ul>

Our Daily Schedule

6:00 a.m.	Morning prayer, take him off machines
6:45 a.m.	Bathe him and brush his teeth
7:00 a.m.	Back brace / Get him dressed
7:30 a.m.	Snack
8:00 a.m.	Ready for pick-up

8:15 a.m.	Bus pick-up
3:50 p.m.	Back home
4:00 p.m.	Homework
4:30 p.m.	Snack
5:00 p.m.	Dinner
5:30 p.m.	Machine
6:00 p.m.	Read
6:30 p.m.	Laydown
8:00 p.m.	Roll over

Final Thoughts

It's simple but please cover your mouth when you cough. People with low or poor immune systems get sick quickly. What you don't understand is, something so simple can really hurt them. So please, cover your mouth when you cough so my child won't have to visit the ER. And be thankful for your healthy child!

5. Highlights

Like I said before, sometimes being in a chair is not all bad. I have had some fun things happen to me and my family, especially when I turned 6 years old. Here are some of my highlights:

My 6th Birthday

It was very good. I loved my birthday party. I had Star Wars, Darth Vader, Storm Trooper and I ate a lot! It was fun drawing on the table and playing with Autumn, one of my best friends. It was a great party.

I really loved my birthday, especially when I got a lot of money, hopefully to buy those red and gold shoes I wanted. We also had a clown who played the paper jams and I played the guitar. The music was really good, like when the DJ played Mindless Behavior.

I really, really loved the food, especially the mac and cheese! Love you Auntie Ellen ☺ Thank you Ms. Anderson for coming to my party! Thank you to Auntie Rhonda and Kenyatta, and Auntie Bridgette for booking us a vacation. I love you all!

May 19th

I was in a concert at school. We had to sing in

front of all those people; but it was fun.

Exercises for Exceptional Children!

My doctor always talks to me about not gaining too much weight and how important it is to get as much exercise as I can. So, last year I made an exercise video for kids in wheelchairs. It is posted on YouTube under the name Lil Torrance. I demonstrated seven Exercises for Exceptional Children that can be done by kids in wheelchairs. They are:

1. Wheelchair Jumping Jacks
2. Wheel Chair Swimming
3. Knee Lifts
4. Wheelchair head rest; up & down
5. Shoulder to ear
6. Toe Taps
7. Hands – open & close

Do each exercise 5 times.

Summer Camp

I finally turned 6 which meant I could go to a camp for kids with SMA and MD. It was great! There were kids there who knew how I felt and what I go through. They had wheelchairs and leg braces just like me. I had no worries.

I was with them for a whole week and it was the best week of my life. We went horseback riding, tree climbing, and riding on motorcycles and to the beach.

Public Speaking

On Thursday July 21, 2011 I spoke at Oakland

Community College. It was my first time public speaking. My cousin attends that school and she wanted me to talk about my disease – SMA Type II. It is a neuro-muscular disease. It is also a progressive disease that affects all of the nerves and muscles in my body and is terminal. I explained to them how I use my power chair and about all of my machines and feeding tubes that I have to have at night.

We talked about how the disease affects my family. I told them about one time when my cousin came over and wanted to play but I could not because I have to get on the machine at a certain time every day. That made me really mad so I just said a prayer and started to sing my church songs and I felt better.

I discussed my fight with the school and how they did not want to give me an aide. They also said I could not take my machines into school because it would take up too much time. My Mom even told them how hard it was to find a school for children with 'exceptions'. And sometimes it is challenging when people don't seem to recognize how they speak to you, or it seems like they are afraid to touch you.

I am involved in the MDA fundraisers such as The Muscle Walk, Fill the Boot, MDA Christmas Party Telethon just to name a few. This year I was nominated for the State of Michigan Goodwill Ambassador for MDA.

Some other speaking events were at Renaissance High School, Menchie's Restaurant, Hockey Town Café, Wayne Westland Fire Department, and MDA staff meeting. I always speak to people about what I have, how I live and how I don't let this disease get to me. I live every day like it's golden.

My Wish Comes True

When my doctor told me about the Make A Wish Foundation, I knew right away what my wish would be; to meet President Barack Obama! It took almost a year but President Obama was not available. My second choice was to meet Mrs. Michelle Obama and we got to do that.

This is the letter Dr. McCormick wrote to Mrs. Michelle Obama to explain the disease:

May 20, 2012

Dear Mrs. Obama:

Thank you very much for your kindness in granting Torrance's wish to "meet with Michelle Obama". As a pediatric neurologist and through my work with the Make A Wish Foundation, I have found that most children opt for a trip to Disney World. Torrance is special. He is articulate, intelligent, charismatic, courageous and wise beyond his years.

Torrance represents a subgroup of muscular dystrophy patients diagnosed with spinal muscular atrophy, whose physical limitations are more than compensated by their intelligence and courage. Many of them will achieve advanced degrees. Like Torrance, each one of my patients is special in that they have the capacity to triumph over adversity. The main obstacles to their success are the lack of public awareness and ultimately, funding to meet their everyday needs. They are handicapped and much of their needs are palliative. As a result, they have become the forgotten society. For every Stephen Hawkins, whose scientific achievements overshadow his physical handicap, there are many children like Torrance, enthusiastically waiting for a chance to fulfill their dreams, in spite of their physical limitations.

Today, you have graciously fulfilled Torrance's long awaited wish. Tomorrow, we as a society have an obligation to allow our children to fulfill their aspirations and dreams. Ultimately, the greatness of our great society is not measured by how we treat the rich, but by the compassion and care that we provide for the disadvantaged. Thank you again for your sensitivity and your awareness displayed for my patient.

Most sincerely,

M. Eileen McCormick, D.O. FAAP

\\\

Our whole family went to Washington D.C. It was my first time on a plane. We went all over the city, to the National Museum, the Pentagon and to the Capitol Building. Dillan was our tour guide through the Pentagon. We stayed at the W Hotel, which is a very nice hotel across the street from the White House. We did not get to go to the Treasury building, so I don't know what that's all about.

It was fun when we got to take pictures with the secret service. Ellie and Sarah were our tour guides. We got to take pictures with the K9 unit. They have a big dog that sniffs out explosives on people and on vehicles. The Secret Service has to protect the president and his family, keeping them safe from the bad people.

Once we got inside the White House, there was a special line that crosses into the White House. (YEAH!) Next we saw the different rooms. The blue room, which is blue, and the red room, which is red, are Mrs. Obama's favorite rooms. We saw the China room, the entertaining room where the huge chandeliers are. Then we toured the kitchen and met the chefs who prepare Mr. and Mrs. Obama's; and the kids, food. Oh yeah, and we met the pastry chef too.

Next we went into the flower shop where they have hundreds of flowers. They were very nice – they gave me a purple flower and I had on purple which is Mrs. Obama's favorite color. We even got to see the 1st family's bowling alley. Mr. Sarah said only guests of the 1st family can play and I was happy when he said "You are guests of the 1st family, you can play!" "Yes!" I said and we toured a couple more rooms.

Then the time finally came when I got to meet her. They took me into this room, then "Here she comes" they said when she came in the room. I smiled from ear to ear. I felt so happy but I couldn't remember the stuff I wanted to tell her, so I asked my mom to remember it in case I forgot.

She was a very nice person. We talked about school and what we were doing for the summer. I liked it when she called me 'old man'. She's beautiful and really, really, really a nice person. I got to meet their dog Bo; he was a really good dog. We talked for a long time then she went to a lunch at the Capitol Building and we went to lunch at the Old Ebbitt Grill.

We even went shopping for souvenirs but I did not like that we had to take those crazy machines.

Thank you Make A Wish for making my wish come true!

My Mom Says

Meeting Mrs. Obama was a special day for all of us. We all took pictures with her and she took several with Torrance. In one of my favorite pictures he is reading the letter from his doctor that describes SMA to Mrs. Obama. Then there is the one where she is saying something funny to Torrance and he is cracking up laughing.

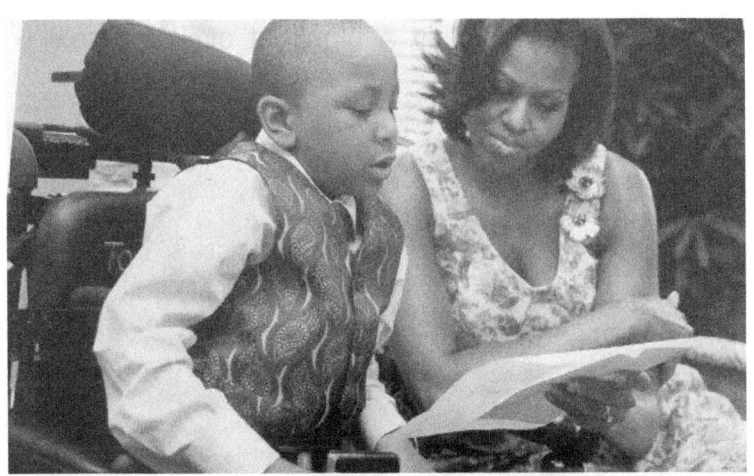

Torrance reading Dr. McCormick's letter to Mrs. Obama. White House photo.

They had a lot of conversation. She thought it was great that he had done an exercise video for Exceptional Kids because they need to exercise too. She asked him what his favorite subject was in school and when she saw his bible, she asked if he always carried it with him. He told her yes. She also signed

Lavonta's bible.

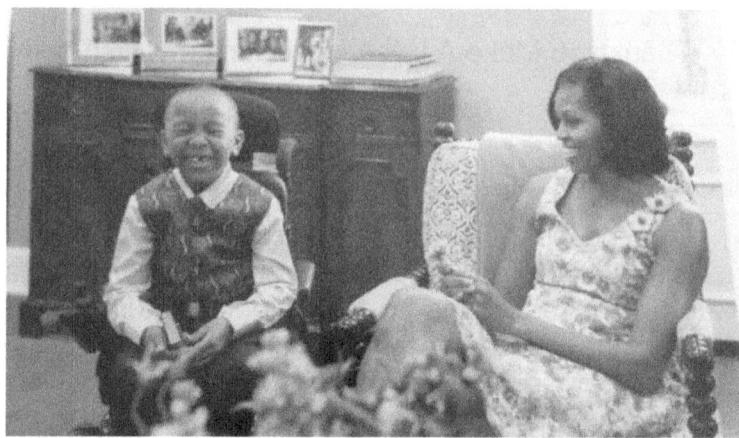

Mrs. Obama makes Torrance laugh, his Bible in hand. White House photo.

This trip was definitely a highlight of Torrance's 6th year.

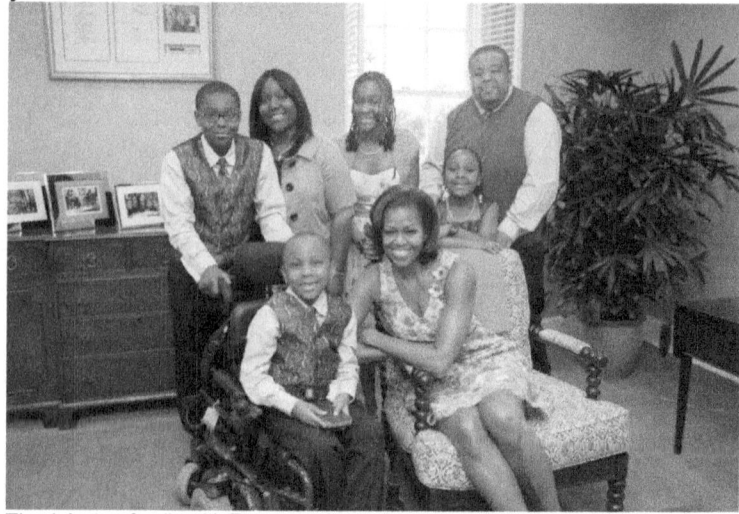

The Johnson family with First Lady Michelle Obama. White House photo.

6. A Hope and a Future

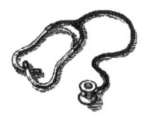

"Talking to People is my Therapy!"

I feel that my calling is to talk to people, young or old it doesn't matter. I talk to them about the disease and how to treat people in wheelchairs with respect. Even people with disabilities should be treated with respect.

Summer Camp

My dream is to have my own summer camp where the key is to have fun, to learn and to build. There would be helpers to help kids with the bathroom and whatever help the kids need. The kids would bring their own power chairs.

There would be tables to do work on, like arts & crafts. The handicap swings will have seatbelts and the handicap slides will have buckles, back support and pillows on the seat so your booty won't get tired. We will be able to play hide and seek, paint, make wooden bird houses, read the bible and have pillow fights. There would also be a reading program.

I would really like to design shoes for kids with the help of one of the big shoe companies. They would only cost $25.00, but would be free if some kids couldn't afford them. We would call them 'Toe Jams' and they would be special shoes for kids who wear braces and come in red and gold or black and white.

You've Got to Have Faith!

To me, faith is something you can't see, but you believe in. It is to believe in God and have faith even in your current situation.

God keeps me in good spirits. When I share my story I want people to have hope and faith. I have faith that a cure for the disease will come and no more people will have to deal with it. Hope to me is that in the future people will not get the disease, but if they do God heals their spirit so they can deal with it. Because if you don't learn how to deal with the disease, your spirit will be down and not where it needs to be for you to have happiness.

I really enjoy gospel music because it fills my spirit with joy and happiness and I feel like dancing. I think of a place where there are no sick people, no disease, no wheelchairs, no machines, no more pain and everyone is happy; everyone is a believer!

I had thought about changing the title of my book because I don't really believe in hate. But I do really believe that one day diseases like Spinal Muscular Atrophy will be wiped out, eliminated – no more! That is my hope and my faith.

MDA Letter

MDA Muscular Dystrophy Association
Fighting Muscle Disease

3300 East Sunrise Drive, Tucson, AZ 85718-3299
Telephone (520) 529-2000 • Fax (520) 529-5300
mda.org • mda@mdausa.org

January 28, 2014

Torrance Johnson

Canton, MI 48187

Dear Torrance:

Congratulations! I just heard you've been selected as MDA's 2014 Michigan Goodwill Ambassador. That's exciting news indeed! We truly appreciate your dedication to spreading our message of help and hope.

During your year as MDA State Goodwill Ambassador, you'll meet generous supporters and represent MDA at many important and fun-filled events. In addition, you'll be helping us gain new friends in our battle against muscle diseases.

Thank you for sharing your story!

Sincerely,

Courtney McEleney

Courtney McEleney
MDA Community Relations Manager

Make a Muscle, Make a Difference®

Torrance Hates SMA

About the Authors

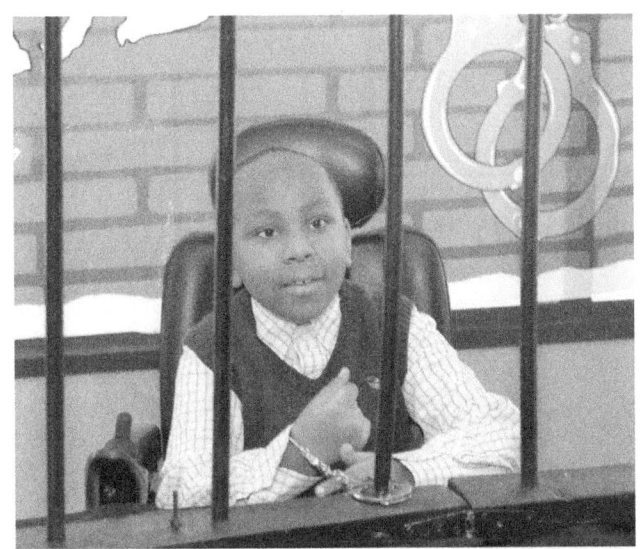

Torrance at the MDA Lock-Up fundraiser in Southfield, MI

Torrance Johnson Jr. was 7 years old when he began writing this book. He is a student at Eriksson Elementary School in Canton, Michigan where he resides with his family. Torrance is a leader in the church youth program and a helper at school. Torrance has been public speaking since age 5 and is the 2014 MDA Goodwill Ambassador for the state of Michigan.

Torrance is available for public speaking events and book-signings. Contact him via his mother, Katrina Johnson at:
Email: Liltoe200six@yahoo.com
FaceBook: Torrance Johnson Jr.
Twitter: @liltoe2006

Torrance Hates SMA

About the Authors

Katrina Johnson

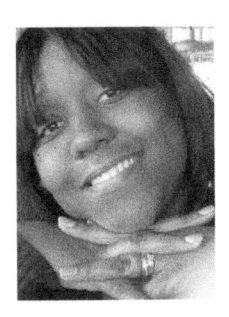

Mrs. Katrina Johnson is married to Torrance Elton Johnson Sr. and is the mother of 4 children. She is young Torrance's primary care giver and is the former owner of New Beginnings Christian Home Day Care.

Katrina has faced numerous challenges in her life such as finding her mother dead in their home when she was just 11 years old. Then there was a diagnosis of ovarian cancer, a stroke (and rehabilitation) and now caring for her son who depends on her to get through his day.

She coined the phrase "Exceptional Children" to describe children who have disabilities like Torrance's. Her life view is that "Embracing one's charitable destination with love, passion, perseverance, commitment and dedication is the only way to fulfill one's remarkable destiny!" And it is impossible to do that without faith.

Co-authoring this book with Torrance was challenging also as it caused her to review many painful parts of his journey. It also gave her many things to be thankful for.

Mrs. Johnson can be reached at:
liltoe200six@yahoo.com or FB Katrina Johnson